a slacker's guide to genetics

A Beginner's Guide to Genetics

william webb

contents

introduction

decoding life: why genetics matter

Welcome to our journey through the fascinating world of genetics. You might be wondering, "Why should I even care about genetics?" Well, let me tell you, it's much more than just a topic in your high school biology class. Genetics is at the core of who we are, shaping our physical appearance, health, and even our personalities.

First of all, genetics helps us understand how traits are passed from parents to their offspring. By studying inheritance patterns, we can better predict the likelihood of certain characteristics in future generations. This knowledge has practical applications, such as guiding the breeding of plants and animals for agriculture, or informing couples about the risks of passing on genetic disorders to their children.

On a larger scale, genetics plays a crucial role in medicine. Genetic research has led to the discovery of many genes responsible for various diseases, which in turn has paved the way for the development of targeted therapies and personalized medicine. Imagine a world where doctors can tailor treatments specifically to your genetic makeup, increasing the chances of successful outcomes and reducing side effects. That's the power of genetics!

But it's not just about health; genetics also sheds light on our evolutionary past. By comparing the DNA of different species, we can uncover fascinating insights into how life on Earth has evolved over millions of years. Genetics allows us to explore the relationships between organisms, revealing our shared ancestry and the unique adaptations that have shaped the living world.

Moreover, genetics is at the forefront of cutting-edge technologies. Genetic engineering has revolutionized fields like agriculture, enabling us to create crops that are more resistant to pests and harsh environmental conditions. And with the advent of gene editing tools like CRISPR-Cas9, we are now able to precisely modify the DNA of organisms, opening up endless possibilities for scientific and medical break-throughs.

But wait, there's more! Genetics also touches on ethical and philosophical questions that challenge our understanding of what it means to be human. As our ability to manipulate DNA grows, so do concerns about the potential consequences. How far should we go in editing the human genome? What are the implications for privacy as genetic information becomes more accessible? Genetics encourages us to reflect on these important issues.

Now that you've got a taste of why genetics is so important, I hope you're as excited as I am to dive into the depths of this fascinating subject. As we unravel the mysteries of DNA, genes, and chromosomes, you'll discover just how much genetics influences our lives and shapes the world around us. Let's get started on this incredible journey, and who knows, maybe you'll find that genetics holds the key to unlocking your own hidden potential!

a brief history of genetics: from peas to dna

Our next stop on this fascinating journey through genetics! Before we dive into the nitty-gritty details of DNA, genes, and chromosomes, let's take a moment to appreciate the milestones that have led us to our current understanding of genetics. From humble peas to the discovery of the double helix, the history of genetics is full of twists and turns that have revolutionized our understanding of life.

A monk and his peas: Gregor Mendel's pioneering work

Our story begins in the mid-19th century with Gregor Mendel, an Austrian monk who laid the foundation for modern genetics. Fascinated by the inheritance of traits in pea plants, Mendel meticulously crossbred different varieties and observed their offspring. Through his experiments, he deduced the fundamental laws of inheritance, which explained how traits are passed down through generations. Mendel's work remained largely unrecognized during his lifetime, but later scientists would come to appreciate its groundbreaking significance.

Chromosomes: The carriers of genetic information

As microscopes improved, scientists began to explore the microscopic world of cells. In the late 1800s and early 1900s, researchers discovered structures called chromosomes, which are located in the cell nucleus. They observed that chromosomes come in pairs and are involved in the process of cell division. This discovery led to the realization that chromosomes play a vital role in the transmission of genetic information.

DNA: The blueprint of life

Fast forward to the 1940s, and researchers were hot on the trail of identifying the molecular basis of heredity. In 1953, the famous duo of James Watson and Francis Crick, building upon the work of Rosalind Franklin and Maurice Wilkins, proposed the now-iconic double helix structure of DNA. They realized that DNA is a long molecule made up of four chemical bases, which together form a code for creating proteins. This discovery was a turning point in genetics, revealing the molecular basis of inheritance and setting the stage for the modern era of genetic research.

The Genetic Code: Deciphering the language of life

With the structure of DNA in hand, scientists in the 1960s began to uncover how genetic information is translated into proteins, the workhorses of the cell. Through a series of brilliant experiments, researchers like Marshall Nirenberg, Har Gobind Khorana, and Sydney Brenner cracked the genetic code, showing how the sequence of DNA bases corresponds to the sequence of amino acids in proteins. This understanding paved the way for exploring the regulation of gene expression and the complex interplay between genes and their products.

The Human Genome Project: Mapping our genetic blueprint

In the late 20th and early 21st centuries, advances in technology allowed scientists to embark on an ambitious mission: sequencing the entire human genome. The Human Genome Project, a massive international collaboration, was completed in 2003, providing researchers with an invaluable resource for understanding the function of our genes and how they contribute to health and disease. This accomplishment marked a new era in genetics, opening up countless possibilities for research and application.

As we continue to explore the world of genetics, we'll build upon this rich history, delving into the details of DNA, genes, and chromosomes, and discovering how they all come together to create the tapestry of life. So buckle up, because we're about to take a thrilling ride into the microscopic world that lies at the heart of our very existence!

navigating the genetic landscape: our goals and guideposts

Now that we've dipped our toes into the fascinating world of genetics, let's talk about what we aim to achieve with this book and how we plan to guide you on this incredible journey. We understand that genetics can seem a bit daunting, but fear not! We've designed this book to be both accessible and engaging, allowing you to explore the wonders of genetics without feeling overwhelmed.

Our primary objective is to provide you with a solid foundation in the core concepts and principles of genetics, tailored to those who are new to the field or simply curious. We'll start with the basics, like the structure and function of DNA, genes, and chromosomes, and gradually build upon these concepts as we delve into topics such as gene expression, inheritance patterns, genetic disorders, and evolution.

But that's not all! We also aim to showcase the incredible applications of genetics in various fields, from agriculture and biotechnology to medicine and personalized healthcare. We'll discuss how genetic engineering and gene editing are revolutionizing our world and explore the ethical dilemmas that these advances present.

Throughout the book, we'll make complex ideas more digestible and approachable. As we progress through the chapters, we encourage you to reflect on the information and consider how genetics influences your own life and the world around you. Our goal is not just to inform but also to inspire curiosity and critical thinking.

In the end, we hope that this book will leave you with a newfound appreciation for the incredible world of genetics and a desire to continue exploring this fascinating field. As we embark on this adventure together, remember that every journey begins with a single step (or, in this case, a single base pair!). So let's get ready to unravel the mysteries of the genetic code and uncover the secrets that lie within the very essence of life.

1 /
the basics of genetics

decoding dna: understanding life's masterplan

NOW THAT WE'VE set the stage, it's time to dive deeper into the star of the show: DNA. This extraordinary molecule is the master architect of life, holding the instructions for constructing and maintaining every living organism on Earth. Let's explore the intricacies of DNA, from its elegant structure to its vital role in the living world.

Structure and components: DNA's building blocks

DNA, short for deoxyribonucleic acid, is a long, twisted ladder-like structure known as the double helix. Its backbone consists of alternating sugar and phosphate molecules, while the rungs are made up of pairs of nitrogenous bases. There are four different bases: adenine (A), thymine (T), cytosine (C), and guanine (G). These bases pair up in a specific manner: A always pairs with T, and C always pairs with G. It's like a molecular dance where each base has its perfect partner!

The genetic code: DNA's language of life

The sequence of bases in DNA forms the genetic code, which serves as a set of instructions for creating proteins, the molecules responsible for carrying out various functions within the cell. Each set of three bases, called a codon, corresponds to a specific amino acid, the building blocks of proteins. With four bases and three-base-long codons, there are 64 possible combinations, which is more than enough to cover the 20 different amino acids found in proteins. Talk about a versatile language!

DNA replication: Copying the blueprint for life

For life to continue and grow, cells must divide, and to do so, they need to make copies of their DNA. During a process called DNA replication, the two strands of the double helix unwind, and special enzymes called DNA polymerases read the original strands while adding complementary bases to create new strands. The end result is two identical DNA molecules, each containing one original and one newly synthesized strand. It's like having a flawless photocopy machine inside each cell!

As we journey further into the realm of genetics, we'll see how this amazing molecule not only serves as life's blueprint but also influences every aspect of our existence. From determining our physical traits to playing a crucial role in our health and well-being, DNA truly is the cornerstone of life. So, let's continue our adventure and discover how DNA's instructions are translated into the proteins that shape our world, one base pair at a time.

genes unleashed: the workhorses of inheritance

It's time to introduce you to the real stars of the genetic show: genes. These tiny, yet mighty, functional units of heredity are the driving force behind the incredible diversity of life on Earth. So, let's roll up our sleeves and delve into the world of genes, from their structure and function to their role in the grand tapestry of inheritance.

What's in a gene? Structure and organization

A gene is a specific segment of DNA that contains the instructions for making a particular protein. Genes are organized within the long, coiled strands of DNA, which are packaged into structures called chromosomes. Each gene has a unique sequence of base pairs, determining its specific function within the cell. It's like a recipe in the cookbook of life, with each gene providing the steps to create a specific dish (or, in this case, a protein).

Express yourself: Turning genes on and off

But genes aren't always active; they need to be turned on, or expressed, at the right time and in the right place. The process of gene expression involves two main steps: transcription, where the DNA sequence of a gene is copied into a molecule called RNA, and translation, where the RNA sequence is used as a template to build a protein. The regulation of gene expression is essential for the proper functioning of cells and the development of organisms. It's like having a well-timed traffic light system within our cells, ensuring everything runs smoothly.

Inheritance at work: Passing genes from generation to generation

Genes are the vehicles through which traits are passed from parents to offspring. When organisms reproduce, their genes are shuffled and combined in various ways, resulting in the unique genetic makeup of each individual. This process, called genetic recombination, is responsible for the incredible diversity of life on Earth. It's like mixing and matching different Lego blocks to create countless unique structures.

chromosomes: the librarians of the genetic world

If genes are the recipes in the cookbook of life, then chromosomes are the librarians that keep everything organized and in order. As we journey further into the realm of genetics, let's explore the role of chromosomes in organizing genetic information and ensuring the proper functioning of our cells.

Structure and composition: Chromosomes' dynamic design

Chromosomes are thread-like structures found within the nucleus of our cells, made up of DNA tightly wrapped around proteins called histones. This compact packaging is essential for fitting the vast amount of genetic information within the tiny confines of the cell nucleus. It's like having a state-of-the-art filing system that can store an entire library's worth of books in a single room.

The numbers game: Human chromosomes and their pairs

Humans have 46 chromosomes, which are arranged in 23 pairs. One chromosome from each pair is inherited from our mother, and the other comes from our father. The first 22 pairs, known as autosomes, are the same in both males and females. The 23rd pair, called the sex chromosomes, determines our biological sex: females have two X chromosomes (XX), while males have one X and one Y chromosome (XY). It's like a chromosomal lottery, with the prize being your unique combination of traits!

Cell division: Chromosomes in action

Chromosomes play a crucial role in the process of cell division. During mitosis, the process of cell division for growth and repair, chromosomes replicate and are then divided equally between two new cells. In meiosis, the process that creates sperm and egg cells, chromosomes are shuffled and divided, resulting in cells with half the number of chromosomes (haploid cells). This ensures that when sperm and egg cells combine during fertilization, the resulting offspring has the correct number of chromosomes. It's like a well-choreographed dance, with chromosomes gracefully moving in perfect harmony.

As we uncover more about the fascinating world of genetics, it's clear that chromosomes play a vital role in organizing and protecting our genetic information. They are the unsung heroes, ensuring that the recipes in our cookbook of life are passed on accurately from one generation to the next.

2 /

the central dogma: from dna to proteins

transcription: the genetic telegram from dna to rna

AS WE DELVE DEEPER into the genetic realm, it's time to explore transcription, the vital process that allows our cells to interpret the genetic code and turn it into something they can use. Think of transcription as a trusty messenger that carries important instructions from the DNA to the rest of the cell. Let's take a closer look at this fascinating process and discover how our cells transform genetic information into RNA.

The initiation: Let the message begin

Transcription begins with a process called initiation, where a group of proteins called transcription factors bind to a specific region of the DNA, known as the promoter. This signals the start of a gene and recruits an enzyme called RNA polymerase, which will do the actual transcription. It's like the starting line of a race, where the runners (RNA polymerases) are ready to begin their journey.

Elongation: Spelling out the message

Once RNA polymerase is bound to the DNA, it starts the elongation process. During this stage, the enzyme reads the DNA template strand, adding complementary RNA nucleotides one at a time. Adenine (A) in DNA pairs with uracil (U) in RNA, while cytosine (C) pairs with guanine (G). It's like a typewriter, carefully crafting the RNA message letter by letter.

Termination: The end of the line

Transcription continues until RNA polymerase reaches a specific sequence in the DNA called the terminator. At this point, the newly formed RNA molecule, called messenger RNA (mRNA), is released from the DNA template, and the RNA polymerase detaches. The mRNA molecule is now ready to be processed and sent on its way to be translated into protein. It's like reaching the finish line of a race, where the message has been successfully relayed.

Transcription is an essential step in the journey from DNA to functional proteins. This remarkable process allows our cells to access and use the genetic information stored within our DNA, setting the stage for the next exciting chapter in the story of life: translation.

translation: the protein assembly line from rna to action

Having explored the fascinating process of transcription, we now venture into the next stage of the genetic journey: translation. This is where the genetic telegram, now in the form of messenger RNA (mRNA), is decoded to produce the proteins that carry out vital functions in our cells. Get ready to witness the incredible assembly line that turns RNA messages into the molecular workforce of life.

The cast of characters: Meet the molecules

Translation requires a team of molecular players, each with a specific role. The star of the show is mRNA, which carries the genetic code from the DNA. Then, we have transfer RNA (tRNA), which brings the right amino acids to the assembly line. Last but not least, we have ribosomes, the cellular factories where proteins are assembled. It's like a well-orchestrated production line, with each member working in harmony.

Initiation: A meeting of molecules

The translation process begins with initiation,

where the ribosome and the mRNA come together. The ribosome binds to the mRNA near a special sequence called the start codon, usually AUG, which signals the beginning of the protein-coding sequence. It's like the curtain rising on a theatrical performance, with the stage set and the actors ready to begin.

Elongation: Building the protein chain

During elongation, tRNA molecules bring their corresponding amino acids to the ribosome, matching the mRNA's codons with their complementary anticodons on the tRNA. The ribosome then links the amino acids together, forming a growing chain that will eventually become the protein. It's like a molecular game of Tetris, with each piece falling into place to create a cohesive structure.

Termination: The grand finale

Translation continues until the ribosome encounters a stop codon on the mRNA, which signals the end of the protein-coding sequence. At this point, the ribosome releases the completed protein and detaches from the mRNA. The protein is now ready to be folded into its final shape and perform its function within the cell. It's like the closing scene of a play, where the actors take their final bow, and the curtain falls.

Translation is the grand finale in the process of turning genetic information into functional proteins.

This intricate dance of molecules, from RNA to protein, showcases the elegance and precision of cellular machinery.

gene regulation: the maestro behind genetic harmony

With the processes of transcription and translation under our belts, it's time to explore the fascinating world of gene regulation. Just like a maestro directing an orchestra, gene regulation ensures that the right genes are expressed at the right time and in the right place, creating a harmonious symphony of cellular activity. Let's dive into the intricacies of gene regulation and discover how our cells maintain balance and control.

The importance of timing: When to express genes

Our cells contain thousands of genes, but not all of them need to be expressed all the time. In fact, many genes are only activated under specific conditions or during particular stages of development. Precise control of gene expression is crucial for proper cellular function and organismal development. It's like having a perfectly timed playlist for every moment of your life.

Turning genes on: Activators and enhancers

Gene expression can be initiated by proteins

called activators, which bind to DNA sequences called enhancers. When an activator protein binds to an enhancer, it helps recruit RNA polymerase to the promoter region of a gene, kickstarting the transcription process. It's like pressing the play button on your favorite song when the mood is just right.

Turning genes off: Repressors and silencers

Conversely, gene expression can be halted by proteins called repressors, which bind to DNA sequences known as silencers. When a repressor protein binds to a silencer, it blocks RNA polymerase from accessing the gene's promoter region, effectively preventing transcription. It's like hitting the pause button on a song that doesn't quite fit the moment.

Fine-tuning gene expression: Epigenetics and other mechanisms

In addition to the activators and repressors, gene expression can also be fine-tuned by a variety of other mechanisms, including epigenetic modifications and small RNA molecules. These layers of regulation add further complexity to the process, ensuring that our cells can adapt and respond to a wide range of signals and conditions. It's like having an extensive array of volume controls, equalizers, and sound effects to create the perfect musical experience.

Gene regulation is the conductor that orchestrates

the symphony of life, ensuring that each gene plays its part at the right time and in the right context. As we continue to explore the fascinating world of genetics, let's celebrate the complexity and harmony that gene regulation brings to the cellular stage, guiding our cells through the intricate dance of life.

3 /
inheritance patterns and genetic disorders

mendelian inheritance: unraveling the genetic tapestry

IT'S time to pay tribute to the father of genetics himself, Gregor Mendel, and his groundbreaking discoveries in the field of inheritance. Mendel's work laid the foundation for our understanding of how traits are passed from one generation to the next. Let's take a step back in time and explore the fascinating principles of Mendelian inheritance.

The pea plant experiment: Mendel's claim to fame

Mendel conducted his famous experiments using pea plants, meticulously crossbreeding them and observing the resulting traits in the offspring. Through his observations, Mendel discovered that specific traits are inherited in a predictable manner. It's like a high-stakes game of genetic poker, where you can predict the odds of getting a particular hand.

The laws of inheritance: Mendel's legacy

From his experiments, Mendel formulated three laws of inheritance that still hold true today: the Law of Dominance, the Law of Segregation, and the Law of Independent Assortment. These laws describe how traits are passed down through generations and how they can combine in different ways. It's like a secret code that unlocks the mysteries of inheritance.

Dominant and recessive traits: The genetic power play

Mendel's work revealed that some traits are dominant, while others are recessive. Dominant traits mask the expression of recessive traits when both are present. For example, if a pea plant has one allele for purple flowers (dominant) and one for white flowers (recessive), it will have purple flowers. It's like a genetic game of rock-paper-scissors, where one trait emerges victorious.

Punnett squares: Predicting genetic outcomes

Using Mendel's laws of inheritance, scientists can predict the likelihood of certain traits appearing in offspring. Punnett squares, named after the geneticist Reginald Punnett, are a simple tool for visualizing these genetic probabilities. By organizing the possible combinations of parental alleles, Punnett squares can help us anticipate the genetic tapestry of future generations. It's like having a crystal ball for genetic predictions.

Mendelian inheritance sheds light on the fascinating patterns of trait inheritance and forms the foundation of modern genetics. As we continue our genetic odyssey, let's remember the pioneering work of Gregor Mendel, whose curiosity and dedication laid the groundwork for our understanding of the beautiful and intricate tapestry of life.

non-mendelian inheritance: when genetics throws a curveball

As we've seen, Mendelian inheritance plays a significant role in our understanding of genetics. However, not all traits follow Mendel's rules. In the realm of non-Mendelian inheritance, things can get a bit more complex and unpredictable. Let's dive into the captivating world of non-Mendelian inheritance and uncover the surprises that lie beyond the traditional rules of genetic transmission.

Incomplete dominance: A genetic compromise

In incomplete dominance, neither allele is completely dominant over the other, resulting in a blended phenotype. For example, when a red-flowered plant and a white-flowered plant are crossed, their offspring may have pink flowers. It's like mixing paint colors, where neither hue dominates, and a new shade is created.

Codominance: Sharing the spotlight

Codominance is a form of non-Mendelian inheritance in which both alleles for a trait are expressed equally in the offspring. A classic example is blood type AB, where both A and B alleles are expressed simultaneously. It's like a duet where both singers harmonize and share the stage equally.

Multiple alleles: More options on the genetic menu

Some traits are determined by more than just two alleles, leading to a broader range of possible phenotypes. One well-known example is human blood type, which can be A, B, AB, or O, depending on the combination of multiple alleles. It's like an ice cream shop with various flavors to choose from, instead of just the classic chocolate and vanilla.

Polygenic traits: The genetic ensemble

Polygenic traits are controlled by multiple genes, each contributing to the overall phenotype. Traits like height, skin color, and eye color are determined by the combined effect of several genes. It's like a choir, where each singer contributes their unique voice to create a harmonious whole.

Epistasis: Genetic teamwork

Epistasis occurs when the expression of one gene influences the expression of another gene. In this case, one gene can mask or modify the effect of another gene, creating a more intricate pattern of inheritance. It's like a team of dancers, where the performance of one dancer can affect the entire choreography.

Non-Mendelian inheritance showcases the beautiful complexity and diversity of genetic transmission. As we continue to unravel the mysteries of genetics, let's celebrate the surprises and curveballs that make the science of inheritance even more fascinating and captivating than we could have ever imagined.

genetic disorders: when dna takes an unexpected turn

Throughout our exploration of genetics, we've seen the incredible harmony and complexity of genetic processes. However, sometimes things don't go quite as planned, and genetic mutations can lead to a range of disorders. In this section, we'll delve into the world of genetic disorders, unraveling the causes and consequences of these conditions, and learning about their impact on individuals and families.

The root of the problem: Genetic mutations

Genetic disorders typically result from mutations or errors in an individual's DNA. These mutations can range from single nucleotide changes to large-scale chromosomal abnormalities. Just like a typo in a recipe can lead to an unexpected dish, mutations can have significant consequences for the affected individual.

Inheritance patterns: How genetic disorders are passed down

Genetic disorders can be inherited in various ways, including autosomal dominant, autosomal recessive, X-linked, and mitochondrial inheritance. Understanding these patterns helps scientists and clinicians predict the likelihood of a disorder appearing in future generations. It's like tracing a family tree to reveal hidden connections and patterns.

Common genetic disorders: A closer look

There are numerous genetic disorders, each with unique symptoms, causes, and inheritance patterns. In this section, we'll explore some of the more common disorders, such as cystic fibrosis, Down syndrome, and hemophilia. By understanding these conditions, we can appreciate the challenges faced by affected individuals and their families, and learn about the ongoing efforts to find treatments and cures.

Diagnosis and treatment: Navigating the road ahead

For individuals with genetic disorders, early diagnosis and appropriate treatment are crucial. Advances in genetic testing and screening have made it possible to identify many disorders before or shortly after birth. While some genetic conditions can be managed through medication or lifestyle changes, others may require more complex interventions. It's like plotting a course through uncharted territory, with each individual's journey being unique and challenging.

The future of genetic medicine: Hope on the horizon

As our understanding of genetics grows, so does the potential for developing innovative treatments and therapies for genetic disorders. From gene therapy to personalized medicine, researchers are working tirelessly to find new ways to address the challenges posed by these conditions. It's like a race against time, with scientists pushing the boundaries of knowledge to improve the lives of those affected by genetic disorders.

Genetic disorders are a poignant reminder of the delicate balance that exists within our DNA. As we continue to explore the vast and intricate world of genetics, let's remember the individuals and families affected by these conditions and celebrate the scientific breakthroughs that offer hope for a brighter future.

4 /

genetic variation and evolution

sources of genetic variation: celebrating nature's diversity

IT'S important to recognize the various sources of genetic variation that make each individual unique. From the subtle differences in our physical features to the diverse abilities and talents that make us who we are, genetic variation is the driving force behind the rich tapestry of life. In this section, we'll explore the key factors that contribute to genetic variation, celebrating the beauty of nature's diverse creations.

Mutation: The spark of variation

Mutations, or changes in DNA sequences, are one of the primary sources of genetic variation. While some mutations can lead to genetic disorders, as we've seen in the previous section, many others are harmless or even beneficial. It's like a game of genetic roulette, where each spin of the wheel brings new and unexpected possibilities.

Sexual reproduction: Mixing it up

Sexual reproduction, which involves the combination of genetic material from two parents, is another significant source of genetic variation. Through processes like meiosis and fertilization, sexual reproduction shuffles the genetic deck, creating unique combinations of alleles in each offspring. It's like a dance of DNA, where each partner contributes their own distinctive moves.

Crossing over: A genetic swap meet

During meiosis, the process that produces sperm and egg cells, chromosomes can exchange genetic material through a process called crossing over. This genetic shuffling creates new combinations of alleles, increasing the potential for variation in the resulting offspring. It's like a friendly game of cards, where players trade their best cards to create the ultimate hand.

Gene flow: The great genetic migration

Gene flow, or the exchange of genetic material between populations, is another important source of genetic variation. Through processes like migration, mating, and hybridization, gene flow can introduce new alleles into a population and promote diversity.

It's like a cultural exchange program, where individuals bring their unique traditions and customs to share with others.

Genetic drift: A random walk through the gene pool

Genetic drift is the random change in allele frequencies within a population over time. This process can lead to the loss or fixation of certain alleles, altering the genetic composition of a population. It's like a game of chance, where the roll of the genetic dice can have significant consequences for future generations.

Genetic variation is the cornerstone of life's incredible diversity. As we continue to explore the wonders of genetics, let's celebrate the myriad factors that contribute to the uniqueness of each individual, and marvel at the boundless creativity of nature's handiwork.

population genetics: decoding the dna of communities

As we've seen, genetic variation is an essential part of the natural world, and understanding how it operates within populations is a fascinating area of study. Enter the realm of population genetics, which explores the distribution and behavior of genetic variation within groups of individuals. In this section, we'll take a closer look at the principles and methods of population genetics and how it helps us understand the complex tapestry of life.

The gene pool: A community's genetic treasure trove

A population's gene pool is the complete collection of genetic information within that group. By studying the gene pool, researchers can gain valuable insights into the genetic health, diversity, and evolutionary history of a population. It's like a library filled with the genetic stories of an entire community, just waiting to be explored.

Hardy-Weinberg equilibrium: A genetic balancing act

The Hardy-Weinberg equilibrium is a foundational principle of population genetics, providing a model for understanding how allele frequencies remain stable across generations, assuming certain conditions are met. This principle helps researchers identify when a population is evolving or experiencing disruptions to its genetic balance. It's like a tightrope walker maintaining their balance, despite the challenges and obstacles they face.

Selection pressures: Nature's way of shaping populations

Selection pressures are the various factors that

influence the survival and reproduction of individuals within a population. From environmental challenges to competition for resources, these pressures can drive evolutionary change and shape the genetic makeup of a population. It's like a game show, where contestants must adapt and overcome various challenges to succeed.

Genetic drift and gene flow: Shifting sands of the gene pool

As we've seen in the previous section, genetic drift and gene flow can have significant effects on the genetic composition of a population. Population genetics helps us understand the consequences of these processes and their impact on genetic diversity and evolutionary change. It's like watching the shifting sands of a desert, where the landscape is constantly changing and evolving.

Conservation genetics: Protecting the genetic heritage of species

Population genetics is also an essential tool in the field of conservation, as it helps researchers identify vulnerable populations and develop strategies to preserve their genetic diversity. By understanding the genetic makeup and dynamics of threatened species, scientists can work to safeguard their future. It's like a team of dedicated guardians, protecting the precious genetic treasures of the natural world.

Population genetics offers a fascinating window into the complex interplay of forces that shape the genetic landscape of communities. As we continue our journey through the world of genetics, let's appreciate the rich insights this field provides, helping us understand and protect the intricate web of life that surrounds us.

evolution and natural selection: the ever-changing dance of life

Genetics is not only about understanding the intricacies of our DNA but also about appreciating the grandeur of the evolutionary process. At the heart of this process lies the concept of natural selection, the driving force that shapes the diversity of life on our planet. In this section, we'll explore the fascinating world of evolution and natural selection, delving into the ways these forces have shaped life through the ages.

1. The theory of evolution: A transformative idea

The theory of evolution, proposed by Charles Darwin and Alfred Russel Wallace, revolutionized our understanding of the natural world. It posits that all species have evolved from common ancestors over vast stretches of time, driven by the process of natural selection. It's like a grand, intricate tapestry, with each thread representing a species, woven together to form the fabric of life.

Natural selection: Survival of the fittest

Natural selection is the process by which certain heritable traits become more common in a population over time, as individuals with these traits are more likely to survive and reproduce. This gradual change in the genetic makeup of a population can lead to the emergence of new species and the extinction of others. It's like a never-ending competition, with contestants constantly striving to outperform one another.

Adaptation: Fine-tuning for survival

Adaptations are the physical or behavioral traits that help an organism survive and reproduce in its environment. Through the process of natural selection, adaptations become more common in a population, as individuals with these traits have a better chance of survival. It's like a toolbox, filled with specialized tools that help organisms tackle the challenges of their environment.

Speciation: The birth of new species

Speciation is the process by which new species emerge from existing populations. This can occur through various mechanisms, such as geographic isolation or changes in mating preferences. As populations evolve and adapt to different environments or selective pressures, they can eventually become distinct species. It's like a family tree branching out, with new members appearing over time.

The fossil record: Unearthing the past

The fossil record provides a window into the history of life on Earth, revealing the evolutionary relationships between species and the changes that have occurred over time. By studying fossils, scientists can piece together the story of our planet's rich and diverse past. It's like a treasure hunt, with each discovery providing valuable clues about the history of life.

Evolution and natural selection are the awe-inspiring forces that have shaped the incredible diversity of life on our planet. As we continue to explore the world of genetics, let's marvel at the wondrous interplay between genes and the environment, and celebrate the ever-changing dance of life that unites us all.

genomics and bioinformatics

genome sequencing: decoding life's instruction manual

IN RECENT YEARS, the field of genetics has taken a giant leap forward with the advent of genome sequencing technologies. These powerful tools have allowed scientists to read and interpret the complete genetic information of organisms, providing unprecedented insights into their biology and evolution. In this section, we'll delve into the exciting world of genome sequencing and explore how this groundbreaking technology is transforming our understanding of life.

A brief history of genome sequencing

The journey of genome sequencing began in the 1970s, with the development of methods to determine the sequence of individual genes. Over the decades, advances in technology and computing power have made it possible to sequence entire genomes, from bacteria to humans. It's like a thrilling detective story, with each new discovery revealing deeper layers of the genetic mystery.

The Human Genome Project: A monumental achievement

The Human Genome Project, completed in 2003, was a landmark international effort to sequence the entire human genome. This remarkable achievement has laid the foundation for countless advances in genetics, medicine, and biology. It's like having a map of our genetic landscape, guiding researchers on a journey of discovery.

Next-generation sequencing: Faster, cheaper, and more powerful

Next-generation sequencing technologies have revolutionized genome sequencing by dramatically increasing throughput and reducing costs. These advancements have made it possible to sequence the genomes of thousands of organisms and individuals, unlocking a treasure trove of genetic information. It's like upgrading from a magnifying glass to a high-powered telescope, providing a clearer and more detailed view of the genetic world.

Personal genomics: A glimpse into our own DNA

With the advent of affordable genome sequencing, personal genomics has emerged as a popular way for individuals to learn about their ancestry, traits, and potential health risks. It's like having a personalized guidebook to our genetic heritage, offering valuable insights into our past, present, and future.

Applications and future directions

Genome sequencing has far-reaching applications, from understanding the genetic basis of diseases to improving crop production and conserving endangered species. As technology continues to advance, we can expect even more exciting developments and discoveries in the field of genomics. It's like standing at the edge of an uncharted frontier, eager to explore the vast potential of this powerful technology.

Genome sequencing has opened up a whole new world of possibilities in the field of genetics, allowing us to delve deeper into the mysteries of life. As we continue our journey through the realm of genetics, let's celebrate the groundbreaking advances in genome sequencing and look forward to the incredible discoveries that lie ahead.

William Webb

functional genomics: deciphering the language of life

While genome sequencing has allowed us to read the genetic information encoded in our DNA, functional genomics takes this one step further by helping us understand the roles and interactions of genes and other elements in the genome. In this section, we'll explore the fascinating field of functional genomics and learn how it's helping us decipher the complex language of life.

What is functional genomics?

Functional genomics is a branch of genetics that seeks to understand the function, regulation, and interaction of genes and other genomic elements. By studying how genes are expressed, regulated, and interact with one another, researchers can gain valuable insights into the underlying mechanisms of life. It's like being a linguist, trying to understand the grammar and syntax of the genetic language.

Transcriptomics: The study of gene expression

Transcriptomics is a subfield of functional genomics that focuses on the study of RNA molecules produced by genes. By analyzing the transcriptome, or the complete set of RNA transcripts in a cell, scientists can learn which genes are active and how their expression is regulated. It's like eavesdropping on a cellular conversation, trying to make sense of the lively chatter.

Proteomics: From genes to proteins

Proteomics is another important branch of functional genomics that deals with the study of proteins, the workhorses of the cell. By examining the structure, function, and interactions of proteins, researchers can gain insights into the complex cellular machinery that drives life. It's like being an engineer, studying the blueprint and components of a sophisticated machine.

Epigenomics: Beyond the DNA sequence

Epigenomics is a rapidly growing area of functional genomics that investigates heritable changes in gene expression and regulation that are not caused by changes in the DNA sequence itself. By studying the epigenome, scientists can uncover the intricate layers of regulation that control gene activity. It's like discovering a hidden code, layered on top of the genetic text, that influences how the story unfolds.

Systems biology: Integrating the pieces of the puzzle

Systems biology is an interdisciplinary approach that combines the insights from functional genomics and other fields to develop a holistic understanding of biological systems. By integrating data from various sources, researchers can build detailed models of cellular processes and uncover the complex interplay between genes, proteins, and other factors. It's like assembling a jigsaw puzzle, with each piece contributing to the bigger picture.

Functional genomics has unlocked new avenues for understanding the complex language of life, revealing the intricate connections and interactions that underlie the biology of living organisms. As we continue to explore the wonders of genetics, let's appreciate the depth and richness of functional genomics, and celebrate its contributions to our ever-growing knowledge of the living world.

bioinformatics: harnessing the power of computers to decode life

The massive amounts of data generated by modern genetic research require sophisticated tools and techniques to analyze, manage, and interpret them. Bioinformatics is the field that addresses this challenge, combining biology, computer science, and statistics to make sense of the complex world of genetics. In this section, we'll explore the fascinating realm of bioinformatics and learn how it helps us unlock the secrets hidden within our DNA.

The emergence of bioinformatics

The birth of bioinformatics can be traced back to

the early days of DNA sequencing, when researchers realized that computational methods were needed to handle and analyze the vast amounts of data being generated. Since then, bioinformatics has grown into a thriving interdisciplinary field, driving advances in genetics, molecular biology, and other life sciences. It's like the perfect fusion of biology and technology, working together in harmony.

Data storage and management

One of the key challenges in bioinformatics is storing and managing the colossal amounts of data generated by genetic research. Various databases and repositories have been developed to store this information, making it accessible to researchers worldwide. It's like building a massive library of genetic knowledge, with each book containing a unique piece of the puzzle.

Sequence alignment and comparison

A fundamental task in bioinformatics is comparing DNA, RNA, or protein sequences to identify similarities and differences. Sequence alignment algorithms are used to find the best way to match sequences, revealing evolutionary relationships, functional similarities, and other biologically relevant information. It's like playing a game of "spot the difference," but with genetic sequences instead of images.

Phylogenetics: Tracing the tree of life

Phylogenetics is the study of evolutionary relationships between organisms, and bioinformatics plays a crucial role in reconstructing these relationships based on genetic data. By analyzing DNA or protein sequences, researchers can build phylogenetic trees that depict the evolutionary history of species. It's like uncovering the intricate branches of the tree of life, showing how all living things are connected through a shared ancestry.

Predictive modeling and machine learning

Bioinformatics also involves the development of predictive models and machine learning algorithms to analyze and interpret complex biological data. These cutting-edge computational methods can help identify genes, predict protein structure and function, and uncover complex patterns in genetic data. It's like teaching a computer to become a skilled genetic detective, solving mysteries hidden within the DNA code.

Bioinformatics has played a pivotal role in the advancement of genetics, providing powerful tools and techniques to tackle the vast amounts of data generated by modern research. As we continue to delve into the wonders of genetics, let's celebrate the incredible contributions of bioinformatics and look forward to the exciting discoveries that lie ahead.

6 /

genetic engineering and biotechnology

techniques in genetic engineering: shaping the genetic future

GENETIC ENGINEERING HAS REVOLUTIONIZED the field of genetics, enabling scientists to directly manipulate the DNA of organisms and harness their potential for various applications. In this section, we'll explore the techniques that have shaped the world of genetic engineering and learn how they've transformed our understanding of genetics and our ability to harness its power.

Recombinant DNA technology

Recombinant DNA technology involves the joining of DNA molecules from different sources to create new genetic combinations. This technique has paved the way for producing genetically modified organisms (GMOs), gene cloning, and the production of recombinant proteins. It's like being a genetic tailor, stitching together bits of DNA to create something new and exciting.

CRISPR-Cas9: A revolutionary gene-editing tool

CRISPR-Cas9 has emerged as a groundbreaking gene-editing technique, allowing scientists to precisely add, remove, or alter specific genes within an organism's DNA. This revolutionary tool has opened up new possibilities in genetic research and holds great promise for the future. It's like having a pair of molecular scissors that can snip and edit the genetic code with incredible precision.

Gene therapy: Treating diseases at their source

Gene therapy is a promising technique that involves the insertion, alteration, or removal of genes within an individual's cells to treat or prevent diseases. By targeting the underlying genetic cause of a disease, gene therapy has the potential to revolutionize medicine and improve the lives of countless patients. It's like being a genetic doctor, prescribing genetic remedies for various ailments.

Genetically modified organisms (GMOs): Engineering life for better or worse

Genetically modified organisms (GMOs) are created by introducing specific genes into an organism's genome to achieve desired traits. While GMOs have led to significant advances in agriculture, medicine, and other fields, they also raise ethical and environmental concerns. It's like playing the role of a genetic architect, designing living beings with new and improved features.

Synthetic biology: Building life from scratch

Synthetic biology is an emerging field that combines genetic engineering with the principles of engineering and computer science. This interdisciplinary approach aims to design and construct new biological systems or redesign existing ones for useful purposes. It's like being a genetic engineer, constructing new forms of life from the ground up.

Genetic engineering techniques have opened up new possibilities and challenges in the world of genetics. As we continue to explore the potential of these powerful tools, let's appreciate their impact on our understanding of life and their potential to shape the future of genetics and biotechnology.

applications in biotechnology: genetics at work in the real world

The fascinating world of genetics isn't just confined to research labs; it has made a significant impact on a wide range of industries through the field of biotechnology. In this section, we'll explore how genetics has been applied to various areas of biotechnology, transforming our lives and improving the world around us.

Agricultural biotechnology: Feeding the world with genetically engineered crops

Agricultural biotechnology has revolutionized modern farming practices through the development of genetically modified (GM) crops. These crops are designed to be more resistant to pests, diseases, and environmental stresses, leading to increased yields and reduced reliance on chemical pesticides. It's like giving plants their own set of superpowers to help them thrive in challenging conditions.

Medical biotechnology: Developing life-saving therapies and vaccines

Genetics has also played a crucial role in the advancement of medical biotechnology. From developing gene therapies and personalized medicine to creating innovative vaccines and diagnostic tools, genetics has revolutionized the way we approach healthcare. It's like having a genetic toolbox that enables us to design better treatments and prevention strategies for a wide range of diseases.

Industrial biotechnology: Sustainable solutions through bioengineering

Industrial biotechnology leverages genetic engineering to produce environmentally friendly and sustainable solutions for various industries. By harnessing the power of microbes and other organisms, industrial biotechnology can produce biofuels, biodegradable plastics, and other valuable products. It's like being a genetic alchemist, transforming simple organisms into powerful allies for a greener future.

Environmental biotechnology: Cleaning up the planet with genetic help

Environmental biotechnology uses genetic engineering to address environmental challenges, such as pollution and waste management. By engineering microorganisms capable of breaking down toxic substances or producing valuable resources from waste, environmental biotechnology offers promising solutions for a cleaner, more sustainable world. It's like creating a team of microscopic superheroes dedicated to saving the planet.

Forensic biotechnology: Solving crimes with genetic clues

The field of forensic biotechnology has revolutionized crime-solving by using genetic information to identify individuals, determine relationships, and even predict physical appearance. From DNA fingerprinting to ancestry analysis, genetics has become an invaluable tool in the pursuit of justice. It's like being a genetic detective, piecing together clues from the tiniest fragments of DNA.

Genetics has made a profound impact on numerous areas of biotechnology, touching nearly every aspect of our lives. As we continue to explore the endless possibilities of genetics, let's appreciate its incredible applications in biotechnology and the ways it has shaped our world for the better.

ethical considerations and future prospects: balancing progress and responsibility

As we delve deeper into the world of genetics and harness its potential, it is essential to address the ethical considerations that arise from our ever-expanding knowledge and capabilities. In this section, we'll explore some of the most pressing ethical issues in genetics and discuss the future prospects of this fascinating field.

Genetic privacy and discrimination

With the increasing availability of genetic testing and data, concerns about genetic privacy and potential discrimination based on genetic information are more relevant than ever. Ensuring that individuals have control over their genetic data and that it isn't used against them is crucial. It's like having a genetic secret that we must protect from falling into the wrong hands.

Designer babies and human enhancement

Advances in genetic engineering raise the possibility of creating "designer babies" or enhancing human abilities through genetic modification. While these prospects hold potential benefits, they also raise ethical questions about the limits of human intervention and the potential consequences of creating genetic "haves" and "have-nots." It's like walking a tightrope between the power of progress and the pitfalls of playing God.

GMOs and environmental impact

While genetically modified organisms (GMOs) offer potential benefits in agriculture and other industries, they also pose ethical concerns related to their impact on the environment, biodiversity, and potential unforeseen consequences. Striking a balance between the advantages of GMOs and their potential risks is essential. It's like trying to find the perfect recipe that balances all the ingredients for a sustainable and prosperous future.

Gene editing and the future of evolution

As gene-editing technologies like CRISPR-Cas9 become more advanced, the potential to alter the course of evolution itself comes into focus. Deciding how and when to use these powerful tools raises ethical questions about our responsibility to future generations and the potential consequences of tampering with the natural order. It's like being handed the keys to the car of evolution, but needing to drive responsibly.

The future of genetics: Exciting prospects and ethical challenges

The field of genetics holds immense potential for improving our lives and addressing global challenges. As we continue to expand our knowledge and capabilities, we must also grapple with the ethical considerations that come with such power. It's like being on the cusp of a brave new world, where the potential for progress is tempered by our responsibility to navigate its challenges wisely.

As we forge ahead into the future of genetics, let's appreciate the incredible potential of this field while remaining mindful of the ethical considerations that accompany our growing capabilities. By balancing progress and responsibility, we can unlock the full potential of genetics to improve our world and the lives of generations to come.

personalized medicine and genomic medicine

pharmacogenetics and pharmacogenomics: personalizing medicine through genetics

IMAGINE a world where medicines are tailored to your unique genetic makeup, ensuring the highest level of efficacy and the lowest risk of side effects. Welcome to the exciting fields of pharmacogenetics and pharmacogenomics! In this section, we'll explore how these disciplines are revolutionizing medicine and paving the way for personalized treatments.

What are pharmacogenetics and pharmacogenomics?

Pharmacogenetics focuses on how individual genetic variations affect a person's response to specific medications, while pharmacogenomics considers the broader picture of how an individual's entire genome influences their response to drugs. It's like comparing a close-up snapshot of a single gene with a panoramic view of the entire genetic landscape.

The role of genetic variations in drug response

Our genes can influence how we metabolize and respond to medications. Genetic variations may affect drug absorption, distribution, metabolism, or even the target site of action. By understanding these genetic factors, we can better predict drug response and personalize treatments. It's like having a genetic cheat sheet to help us choose the right medicine for each person.

Genotyping and gene panels for drug response

Genotyping and gene panels are techniques used to analyze specific genetic variations associated with drug response. These tests can help healthcare providers determine the most appropriate medications and dosages for patients, reducing the risk of adverse effects and improving treatment outcomes. It's like having a genetic crystal ball to guide us in our medical decision-making.

Personalized medicine: Tailoring treatments to your genes

By incorporating genetic information into health-care decisions, personalized medicine aims to optimize treatments for each individual. This approach can lead to more effective therapies, fewer side effects, and reduced trial-and-error in prescribing medications. It's like having a custom-tailored suit, designed to fit your unique genetic profile.

Future prospects and challenges in pharmacogenetics and pharmacogenomics

As research continues to advance our understanding of genetics and drug response, the potential for pharmacogenetics and pharmacogenomics to revolutionize medicine grows. However, challenges remain in implementing these techniques in clinical practice, such as the need for standardized testing, education for healthcare providers, and addressing ethical considerations. It's like embarking on a thrilling journey, with hurdles to overcome along the way.

Pharmacogenetics and pharmacogenomics hold the promise of transforming medicine by making it more personalized, efficient, and safe. As we continue to unravel the mysteries of our genes and their influence on drug response, let's embrace the potential of these fields to shape the future of healthcare and improve the lives of countless individuals.

genetic testing and counseling: navigating the world of genetics together

Diving into the world of genetics can feel a bit like exploring an uncharted ocean. Genetic testing and counseling are like trusted guides, helping you navigate these waters and make informed decisions about your health and the health of your family. In this section, we'll explore the role of genetic testing and counseling in understanding and managing genetic information.

1. Genetic testing: A window into your DNA

Genetic testing involves analyzing an individual's DNA to identify specific genetic variants associated with certain health conditions or traits. From prenatal screening to carrier testing, genetic testing offers valuable insights into your genetic makeup, providing a roadmap for informed healthcare decisions.

1. Types of genetic tests

There are several types of genetic tests, each with its purpose and application. These include diagnostic testing, carrier testing, prenatal and newborn screening, and predictive and pre-symptomatic testing. It's like having an assorted toolbox of tests, each designed to answer specific questions about your genes.

Interpreting genetic test results

Genetic test results can be complex and sometimes challenging to understand. They may provide information about the likelihood of developing a certain condition, the severity of a disease, or even insights into ancestry and family history. Like interpreting a cryptic treasure map, understanding these results requires knowledge, expertise, and context.

Genetic counseling: Guiding you through the genetic maze

Genetic counselors are specially trained healthcare professionals who help individuals and families understand their genetic test results and make informed decisions. They can provide guidance on appropriate testing options, explain the implications of test results, and offer support for those facing difficult choices. Think of them as the friendly sherpa guiding you through the complex world of genetics.

The role of genetic counseling in healthcare

Genetic counseling plays a crucial role in healthcare by helping patients and healthcare providers navigate the rapidly evolving field of genetics. It aids in informed decision-making, promotes risk assessment and management, and fosters communication between patients, families, and healthcare teams. It's like the glue that holds together the many moving parts of genetics and healthcare.

As we continue to uncover the secrets of our genetic code, genetic testing and counseling will play an increasingly vital role in healthcare. By working together with healthcare professionals and making informed decisions about our genetic information, we can forge a path towards a healthier and more informed future. Embrace the adventure and let genetic testing and counseling be your compass.

gene therapy and regenerative medicine: a new frontier in healing

Welcome to the fascinating realm of gene therapy and regenerative medicine, where science fiction is becoming reality. In this section, we'll explore the cutting-edge technologies that are revolutionizing the way we approach health and healing.

Gene therapy: Correcting genetic errors

Gene therapy involves altering the genes within an individual's cells to treat or prevent disease. By correcting faulty genes or providing functional copies of missing or damaged genes, gene therapy has the potential to address the root cause of many genetic conditions. It's like fixing the typos in the instruction manual that is our DNA.

Methods of gene delivery

Delivering new or corrected genes to cells can be accomplished through various methods, including viral and non-viral vectors. These tiny molecular vehicles act like delivery trucks, carrying the genetic cargo to its destination within the cell. Each method has its advantages and challenges, and choosing the right vehicle is essential for successful gene therapy.

Regenerative medicine: Healing from within

Regenerative medicine focuses on repairing, replacing, or regenerating damaged tissues and organs using our body's natural healing abilities. This approach includes techniques such as stem cell therapy, tissue engineering, and the use of biomaterials. It's like harnessing the superpowers of our own cells to heal and restore our bodies.

Stem cell therapy: The cellular multitaskers

Stem cells are unique cells with the potential to develop into many different cell types in the body. They can serve as a repair system by replenishing damaged tissues and regenerating entire organs. From treating degenerative diseases to regrowing lost limbs, stem cell therapy offers a world of possibilities for healing and restoration.

Ethical and safety considerations

As with any groundbreaking medical technology, gene therapy and regenerative medicine face ethical and safety concerns. Balancing the potential benefits with the risks of unintended consequences, such as immune reactions or off-target genetic changes, requires careful consideration and ongoing research. It's like walking a tightrope, trying to maintain a balance between progress and caution.

As we venture into the exciting world of gene therapy and regenerative medicine, the possibilities for healing and restoration seem almost limitless. These pioneering technologies offer hope for a future where genetic diseases and debilitating conditions can be addressed at their source, transforming the lives of countless individuals.

conclusion

the future of genetics: unlocking the potential of our genetic code

AS WE STAND at the precipice of a new era in genetics, we can't help but marvel at the extraordinary potential that lies within our DNA. In this final section, we'll take a glimpse into the not-so-distant future of genetics and explore the incredible possibilities that await us as we unlock the secrets of our genetic code.

Personalized medicine: Tailoring treatments to your genes

As our understanding of genetics deepens, we'll move toward a future where medical treatments are tailored to our individual genetic profiles. Personalized medicine will allow doctors to prescribe medications and therapies based on each person's unique genetic makeup, increasing the effectiveness of treatments and reducing side effects. It's like having a custom-made suit, tailored precisely to fit you.

Designer babies: The ethics of genetic engineering

The ability to edit our genes raises ethical questions about the potential for "designer babies," where parents could select specific traits for their children. While this technology could prevent the transmission of genetic diseases, it also raises concerns about eugenics and societal inequalities. We must tread carefully as we navigate the uncharted waters of genetic engineering.

Synthetic biology: Building life from scratch

Imagine being able to create entirely new organisms or even design living machines using genetic building blocks. Synthetic biology seeks to do just that, by designing and constructing new biological systems or reprogramming existing ones for specific purposes. From biofuels to pollution-eating microbes, the potential applications are both exciting and mind-boggling.

The genetics of aging: Unlocking the fountain of youth

Our genes hold the key to understanding the aging process and the factors that contribute to age-related diseases. As we delve deeper into the genetics of aging, we may discover ways to extend our lifespans, improve our quality of life, and perhaps even unlock the secret to the fountain of youth. Who wouldn't want to sip from that elixir?

The unknown: Embracing the mysteries of our genetic code

As we continue to explore the vast complexities of our genetic code, we are bound to encounter surprises and challenges along the way. The future of genetics holds untold mysteries, and as we unlock these secrets, we may uncover new possibilities we never even dreamed of. It's like embarking on the greatest adventure of all time, with each new discovery opening up a world of possibilities.

The future of genetics promises to be a thrilling and transformative journey, one that will reshape our understanding of ourselves and the world around us. As we unlock the potential of our genetic code, we'll undoubtedly face challenges and ethical dilemmas, but the promise of a brighter, healthier future for all of humanity is a quest worth pursuing.

the ripple effect: how genetics influences society and individuals

As we've explored the fascinating world of genetics, it's clear that our understanding of this field doesn't merely reside in the pages of a textbook or within the walls of a laboratory. In fact, the impact of genetics stretches far beyond that, touching every aspect of our lives and the society in which we live. In this section, we'll delve into the broader implications of genetics on both individuals and society as a whole.

Health and medicine: A new frontier of possibilities

The impact of genetics on healthcare has been nothing short of revolutionary. From personalized medicine to gene therapy, our growing understanding of genetics is transforming the way we diagnose, treat, and even prevent diseases. This has led to more targeted and effective treatments, better patient outcomes, and an improved quality of life for countless individuals.

The influence on our identities: Nature vs. nurture

Genetics plays a significant role in shaping our identities, from physical traits to predispositions to certain health conditions. As we continue to unravel the complex interplay between our genes and the environment, we gain a deeper understanding of ourselves and what makes us unique. This knowledge can empower individuals to make informed decisions about their health and lifestyle choices.

Legal and ethical considerations: Balancing innovation with responsibility

As genetic technologies advance, they inevitably raise legal and ethical questions. From patenting genes to the use of genetic information in insurance and employment, society must grapple with these complex issues to ensure that the benefits of genetic research are realized while safeguarding the rights and privacy of individuals.

Social dynamics: Understanding the role of genetics in diversity and inequality

Our genetic makeup contributes to the rich tapestry of human diversity, but it can also be a source of inequality and discrimination. Recognizing the role of genetics in shaping social dynamics is crucial for promoting tolerance, understanding, and acceptance in our society. Knowledge, as they say, is power, and understanding our genetic heritage can empower us to break down barriers and foster unity.

Education and public awareness: Demystifying genetics for all

Genetic literacy is essential for individuals to navigate the increasingly complex world of genetic information and make informed decisions about their health and wellbeing. By fostering a greater understanding of genetics, we can help demystify this often-misunderstood field and ensure that its benefits are accessible to everyone, regardless of their background or level of expertise.

The far-reaching impact of genetics on society and individuals underscores the importance of this field in shaping our world. By embracing the knowledge and potential that genetics offers, we can harness its power for the greater good and create a brighter future for all. As we continue to explore the fascinating world of genetics, let's remember that its influence extends far beyond the lab, touching the lives of each and every one of us in myriad ways.

igniting the spark: fostering curiosity and further exploration in genetics

Throughout this book, we've journeyed together through the captivating world of genetics, and it's our hope that this adventure has piqued your curiosity and inspired you to delve even deeper into this fascinating field. In this final section, we'll discuss ways to encourage further exploration and ignite your passion for genetics, keeping the fire of curiosity alive and well.

Lifelong learning: Embrace the student within

Remember, you don't need to be a scientist to appreciate and explore genetics. Lifelong learning is essential to keeping our minds sharp and fostering a sense of wonder. Look for educational resources, such as online courses, podcasts, and documentaries, to continue expanding your knowledge of genetics and related fields.

Engage with the scientific community: Connect and contribute

Joining local or online groups, attending conferences, and engaging with scientists on social media platforms can provide valuable insights and keep you informed about the latest developments in genetics. Engaging with the scientific community is not only a great way to stay current but also offers opportunities to contribute to the conversation and perhaps even collaborate on research projects.

Citizen science: Making a difference in the world of genetics

Citizen science projects, where members of the public can contribute to scientific research, are an excellent way to get involved in genetics without formal training. These projects often involve collecting data or analyzing genetic information, allowing you to contribute to cutting-edge research while deepening your understanding of genetics.

Inspire the next generation: Share your passion for genetics

Sharing your enthusiasm for genetics with others, especially younger generations, can help foster a love of science and inspire future geneticists. Volunteer at local schools or science events, mentor students interested in genetics, or simply share your knowledge with friends and family. By sparking the curiosity of others, you can help create a more scientifically literate and engaged society.

As we close this chapter on our journey through the world of genetics, remember that this is just the beginning of your exploration. The field of genetics is constantly evolving, and there is always more to learn and discover. Embrace the spirit of curiosity, and let it guide you through a lifelong adventure in the captivating realm of genetics.

glossary

decoding the language of genetics: key terms and concepts

THROUGHOUT OUR JOURNEY into the world of genetics, we've encountered numerous terms and concepts that might have been unfamiliar at first. As we wrap up our exploration, let's take a moment to review some of these key terms and concepts in genetics, solidifying our understanding and helping us navigate future conversations and discoveries with confidence.

1. Allele: An alternative form of a gene that arises due to mutation and is found at the same place on a chromosome.

2. Chromosome: A thread-like structure found in the nucleus of cells, composed of DNA and proteins, which carries genetic information in the form of genes.

3. DNA (Deoxyribonucleic Acid): The molecule that carries the genetic instructions for the development, functioning, growth, and reproduction of all known living organisms and many viruses.

4. Gene: A segment of DNA that contains the instructions for building one or more molecules (usually proteins) that help the body function.

5. Genotype: The genetic makeup of an individual organism, consisting of the specific combination of alleles it carries for a particular trait.

6. Phenotype: The physical and observable characteristics of an organism resulting from the interaction of its genotype with the environment.

7. Homozygous: Having two identical alleles for a particular gene.

8. Heterozygous: Having two different alleles for a particular gene.

9. Dominant: An allele that determines the phenotype of an organism, even when another (recessive) allele is present.

10. Recessive: An allele that is only expressed in the phenotype if the dominant allele is not present.

11. Mutation: A change in the DNA sequence that can lead to differences in the structure or function of a gene or its products.

12. Genetic recombination: The process by which genetic material is exchanged between two different chromosomes during the formation of reproductive cells, creating new combinations of genes.

13. Transcription: The process by which the information in a DNA molecule is copied into a complementary RNA molecule.

14. Translation: The process by which the information in an RNA molecule is used to synthesize a protein.

15. Gene regulation: The process by which cells control the amount and timing of gene expression, often in response to changes in the environment or developmental cues.

With these key terms and concepts firmly in mind, you'll be well-equipped to continue your exploration of genetics and engage in informed discussions with other enthusiasts or professionals. Remember, the language of genetics is always evolving, so stay curious and keep learning to stay up-to-date in this dynamic field.

appendices

expanding your genetic horizons: recommended resources

DIVING into the world of genetics can be both exciting and challenging. To help you continue your learning journey and satisfy your growing curiosity, we've compiled a list of additional resources that will guide you towards a deeper understanding of genetics. These resources encompass various formats, so you can choose the ones that best suit your learning style and interests.

Books:

- "The Selfish Gene" by Richard Dawkins
- "The Gene: An Intimate History" by Siddhartha Mukherjee

- "Genome: The Autobiography of a Species in 23 Chapters" by Matt Ridley

Online Courses:

- Coursera: "Introduction to Genetics and Evolution" by Duke University
- edX: "Principles of Evolution, Ecology and Behavior" by Yale University
- Khan Academy: Genetics and Heredity lessons

Podcasts:

- "Genetics Unzipped" by Genetics Society
- "The Naked Genetics Podcast" by The Naked Scientists
- "The Beagle Has Landed" by Genetics Society of America

YouTube Channels:

- iBiology: A collection of high-quality biology talks and lectures by leading scientists.
- Bozeman Science: Educational videos on biology, chemistry, physics, and more,

created by science educator Paul Andersen.

- The Amoeba Sisters: Engaging, animated videos on various biology topics, including genetics.

Websites and Blogs:

- National Human Genome Research Institute (NHGRI): A comprehensive resource for information on genetics, genomics, and related fields.
- DNA Learning Center: A wealth of educational resources, including animations, virtual labs, and more.
- Genetics Home Reference: A consumer-friendly guide to understanding genetic conditions, genes, and chromosomes.

Armed with these resources, you can confidently embark on your own personal journey to learn even more about genetics. Remember, the field of genetics is vast and ever-evolving, so there's always more to discover. Happy exploring, and may your thirst for knowledge be forever quenched by the fascinating world of genetics!

giants of genetics: celebrating renowned researchers

Throughout the history of genetics, numerous scientists have made groundbreaking discoveries that have shaped our understanding of heredity, molecular biology, and evolution. In this section, we will pay homage to some of the most notable figures in the field of genetics. Let's raise a metaphorical glass to these brilliant minds!

1. Gregor Mendel: Known as the "Father of Genetics," Mendel's work on pea plants laid the foundation for the laws of inheritance. His meticulous research and observations led to the discovery of dominant and recessive traits, which are now fundamental concepts in genetics.

2. Rosalind Franklin: An unsung hero, Franklin's work on X-ray crystallography was crucial in revealing the double helix structure of DNA. Unfortunately, her contribution was largely unrecognized during her lifetime, but her legacy as a pioneering scientist lives on.

3. James Watson and Francis Crick: This dynamic duo is famous for proposing the

double helix structure of DNA, which earned them the Nobel Prize in Physiology or Medicine in 1962. Their discovery revolutionized our understanding of genetics and paved the way for countless advances in molecular biology.

4. Barbara McClintock: A trailblazing cytogeneticist, McClintock's groundbreaking research on maize chromosomes led to the discovery of "jumping genes" or transposable elements. Her work earned her the Nobel Prize in Physiology or Medicine in 1983, making her the first woman to win the prestigious award unshared.

5. Eric Lander: A prominent figure in modern genetics, Lander played a significant role in the Human Genome Project, which sequenced the entire human genome. He has since continued to contribute to the field through his research on genomics and human disease.

6. Jennifer Doudna and Emmanuelle Charpentier: These two remarkable scientists were awarded the Nobel Prize in Chemistry in 2020 for their development of the CRISPR-Cas9 gene-editing technology.

This groundbreaking tool has revolutionized the field of genetics and holds great promise for the future of medicine and biotechnology.

As we continue to explore the complex world of genetics, we must not forget to celebrate the scientists who have made it all possible. Their dedication, curiosity, and ingenuity have paved the way for future generations to build upon their remarkable discoveries. Cheers to these exceptional individuals and their contributions to the field of genetics!